Marijuana

Table of Contents

Marijuana

Letter From the Director

What is marijuana?

What is the scope of marijuana use in the United States?

What are marijuana effects?

How does marijuana produce its effects?

Does marijuana use affect driving?

Is marijuana addictive?

What are marijuana's long-term effects on the brain?

Is marijuana a gateway drug?

How does marijuana use affect school, work, and social life?

Is there a link between marijuana use and psychiatric disorders?

What are marijuana's effects on lung health?

What are marijuana's effects on other aspects of physical health?

Is marijuana safe and effective as medicine?

What are the effects of secondhand exposure to marijuana smoke?

Can marijuana use during and after pregnancy harm the baby?

Available Treatments for Marijuana Use Disorders

Where can I get further information about marijuana?

References

Letter From the Director

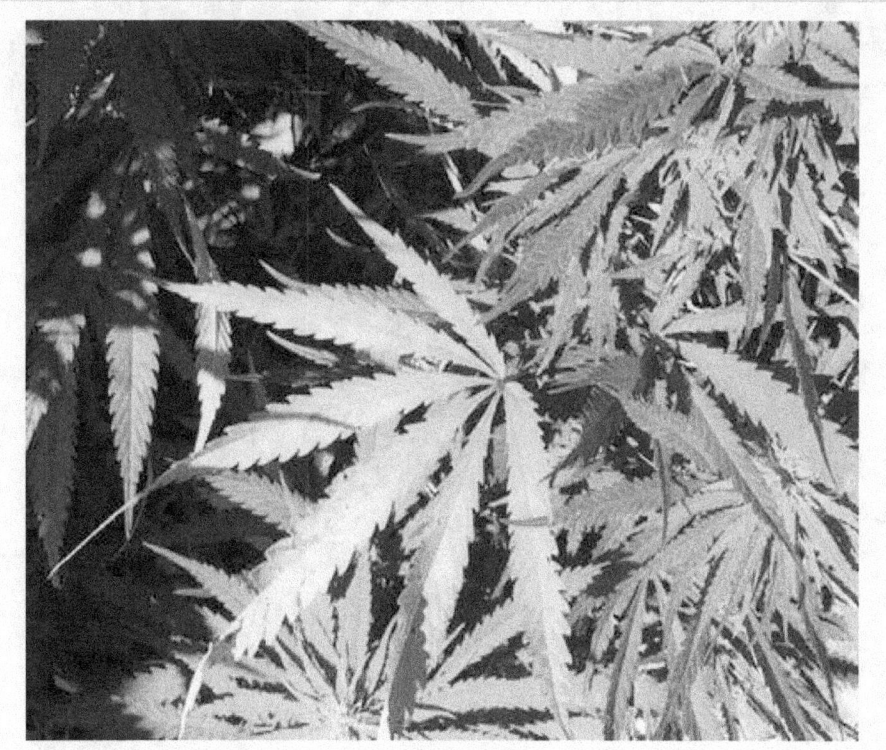
Photo by the NIDA

Changes in marijuana policies across states legalizing marijuana for medical and/or recreational use suggest that marijuana is gaining greater acceptance in our society. Thus, it is particularly important for people to understand what is known about both the adverse health effects and the potential therapeutic benefits linked to marijuana.

Because marijuana impairs short-term memory and judgment and distorts perception, it can impair performance in school or at work and make it dangerous to drive. It also affects brain systems that are still maturing through young adulthood, so regular use by teens may have negative and long-lasting effects on their cognitive development, putting them at a competitive disadvantage and possibly interfering with their well-being in other ways. Also, contrary to popular belief, marijuana can be addictive, and its use during adolescence may make other forms of problem use or addiction more likely.

Whether smoking or otherwise consuming marijuana has therapeutic benefits that outweigh its health risks is still an open question that science has not resolved. Although many states now permit dispensing marijuana for medicinal purposes and there is mounting anecdotal evidence for the efficacy of marijuana-derived compounds, the U.S. Food and Drug Administration has not approved "medical marijuana." However, safe medicines based on cannabinoid chemicals derived from the marijuana plant have been available for decades and more are being developed.

This Research Report is intended as a useful summary of what the most up-to-date science has to say about marijuana and its effects on those who use it at any age.

Nora D. Volkow, M.D.
Director
National Institute on Drug Abuse

See Also:

- Message from the NIDA Director - Marijuana's Lasting Effects on the Brain, (March 2013)

What is marijuana?

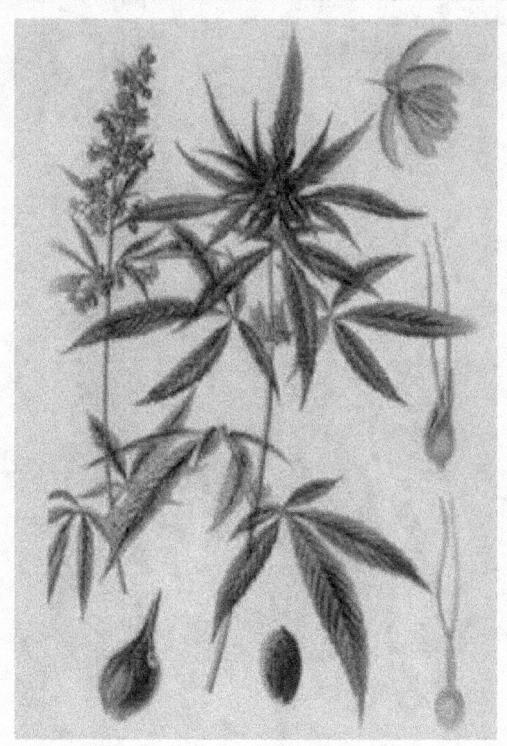
Image by ©iStock.com/nicoolay

Marijuana—also called *weed, herb, pot, grass, bud, ganja, Mary Jane*, and a vast number of other slang terms—is a greenish-gray mixture of the dried flowers of *Cannabis sativa*. Some people smoke marijuana in hand-rolled cigarettes called *joints*; in pipes, water pipes (sometimes called *bongs*), or in *blunts* (marijuana rolled in cigar wraps).[1] Marijuana can also be used to brew tea and, particularly when it is sold or consumed for medicinal purposes, is frequently mixed into foods (*edibles*) such as brownies, cookies, or candies. Vaporizers are also increasingly used to consume marijuana. Stronger forms of marijuana include sinsemilla (from specially tended female plants) and concentrated resins containing high doses of marijuana's active ingredients, including honeylike *hash oil*, waxy *budder*, and hard amberlike *shatter*. These resins are increasingly popular among those who use them both recreationally and medically.

The main *psychoactive* (mind-altering) chemical in marijuana, responsible for most of the intoxicating effects that people seek, is *delta-9-tetrahydrocannabinol* (THC). The chemical is found in resin produced by the leaves and buds primarily of the female cannabis plant. The plant also contains more than 500 other chemicals, including more than 100 compounds that are chemically related to THC, called *cannabinoids*.[2]

What is the scope of marijuana use in the United States?

Marijuana is the most commonly used illicit drug (22.2 million people have used it in the past month) according to the 2015 National Survey on Drug Use and Health.[3] Its use is more prevalent among men than women—a gender gap that widened in the years 2007 to 2014.[4]

Marijuana use is widespread among adolescents and young adults. According to the Monitoring the Future survey—an annual survey of drug use and attitudes among the Nation's middle and high school students—most measures of marijuana use by 8th, 10th, and 12th graders peaked in the mid-to-late 1990s and then began a period of gradual decline through the mid-2000s before levelling off. Most measures showed some decline again in the past 5 years. Teens' perceptions of the risks of marijuana use have steadily declined over the past decade, possibly related to increasing public debate about legalizing or loosening restrictions on marijuana for medicinal and recreational use. In 2016, 9.4 percent of 8th graders reported marijuana use in the past year and 5.4 percent in the past month (current use). Among 10th graders, 23.9 percent had used marijuana in the past year and 14.0 percent in the past month. Rates of use among 12th graders were higher still: 35.6 percent had used marijuana during the year prior to the survey and 22.5 percent used in the past month; 6.0 percent said they used marijuana daily or near-daily.[5]

Medical emergencies possibly related to marijuana use have also increased. The Drug Abuse Warning Network (DAWN), a system for monitoring the health impact of drugs, estimated that in 2011, there were nearly 456,000 drug-related emergency department visits in the United States in which marijuana use was mentioned in the medical record (a 21 percent increase over 2009). About two-thirds of patients were male and 13 percent were between the ages of 12 and 17.[6] It is unknown whether this increase is due to increased use, increased *potency* of marijuana (amount of THC it contains), or other factors. It should be noted, however, that mentions of marijuana in medical records do not necessarily indicate that these emergencies were directly related to marijuana intoxication.

What are marijuana effects?

When marijuana is smoked, THC and other chemicals in the plant pass from the lungs into the bloodstream, which rapidly carries them throughout the body to the brain. The person begins to experience effects almost immediately (see "How does marijuana produce its effects?"). Many people experience a pleasant euphoria and sense of relaxation. Other common effects, which may vary dramatically among different people, include heightened sensory perception (e.g., brighter colors), laughter, altered perception of time, and increased appetite.

If marijuana is consumed in foods or beverages, these effects are somewhat delayed—usually appearing after 30 minutes to 1 hour—because the drug must first pass through the digestive system. Eating or drinking marijuana delivers significantly less THC into the bloodstream than smoking an equivalent amount of the plant. Because of the delayed effects, people may inadvertently consume more THC than they intend to.

Pleasant experiences with marijuana are by no means universal. Instead of relaxation and euphoria, some people experience anxiety, fear, distrust, or panic. These effects are more common when a person takes too much, the marijuana has an unexpectedly high potency, or the person is inexperienced. People who have taken large doses of marijuana may experience an acute psychosis, which includes hallucinations, delusions, and a loss of the sense of personal identity. These unpleasant but temporary reactions are distinct from longer-lasting psychotic disorders, such as schizophrenia, that may be associated with the use of marijuana in vulnerable individuals. (See "Is there a link between marijuana use and psychiatric disorders?")

Although detectable amounts of THC may remain in the body for days or even weeks after use, the noticeable effects of smoked marijuana generally last from 1 to 3 hours, and those of marijuana consumed in food or drink may last for many hours.

How does marijuana produce its effects?

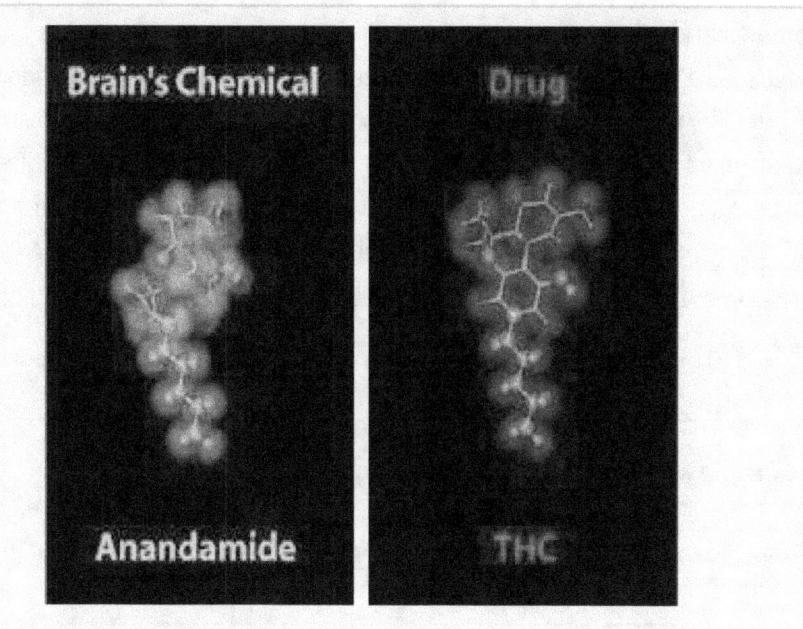

Image by the NIDA
THC's chemical structure is similar to the brain chemical anandamide. Similarity in structure allows drugs to be recognized by the body and to alter normal brain communication.

THC's chemical structure is similar to the brain chemical *anandamide*. Similarity in structure allows the body to recognize THC and to alter normal brain communication.

Endogenous cannabinoids such as anandamide (see figure) function as *neurotransmitters* because they send chemical messages between nerve cells (*neurons*) throughout the nervous system. They affect brain areas that influence pleasure, memory, thinking, concentration, movement, coordination, and sensory and time perception. Because of this similarity, THC is able to attach to molecules called *cannabinoid receptors* on neurons in these brain areas and activate them, disrupting various mental and physical functions and causing the effects described earlier. The neural communication network that uses these cannabinoid neurotransmitters, known as the *endocannabinoid system*, plays a critical role in the nervous system's normal functioning, so interfering with it can have profound effects.

For example, THC is able to alter the functioning of the hippocampus (see "Marijuana, Memory, and the Hippocampus") and orbitofrontal cortex, brain areas that enable a person to form new memories and shift his or her attentional focus. As a result, using marijuana causes impaired thinking and interferes with a person's ability to learn and perform complicated tasks. THC also disrupts functioning of the cerebellum and basal ganglia, brain areas that regulate balance, posture, coordination, and reaction time. This is the reason people who have used marijuana may not be able to drive safely (see "Does marijuana use affect driving?") and may have problems playing sports or engaging in other physical activities.

> People who have taken large doses of the drug may experience an acute psychosis, which includes hallucinations, delusions, and a loss of the sense of personal identity.

THC, acting through cannabinoid receptors, also activates the brain's reward system, which includes regions that govern the response to healthy pleasurable behaviors such as sex and eating. Like most other drugs that people misuse, THC stimulates neurons in the reward system to release the signaling chemical *dopamine* at levels higher than typically observed in response to natural stimuli. This flood of dopamine contributes to the pleasurable "high" that those use who recreational marijuana seek.

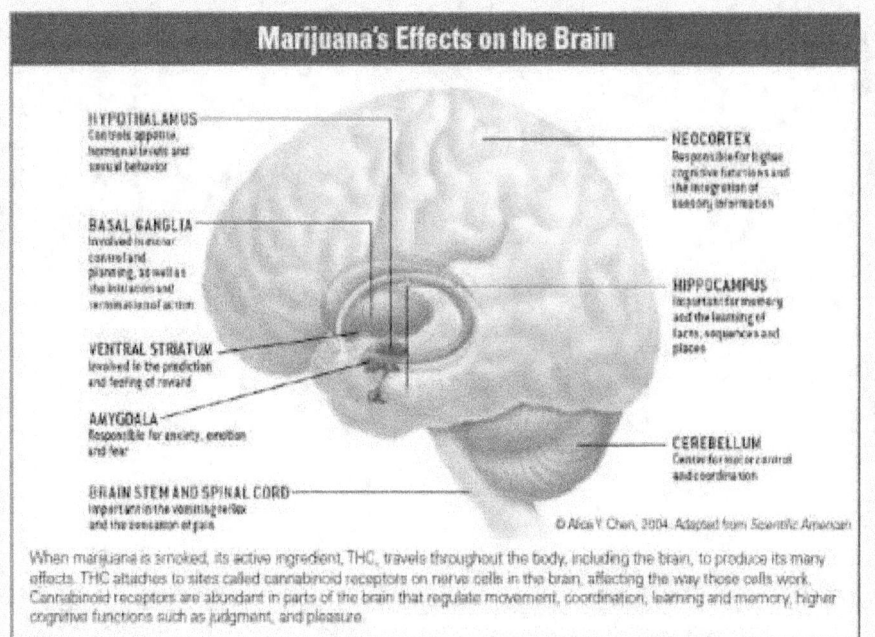

Diagram showing different parts of the brain and describing marijuana's effects on the brain

Does marijuana use affect driving?

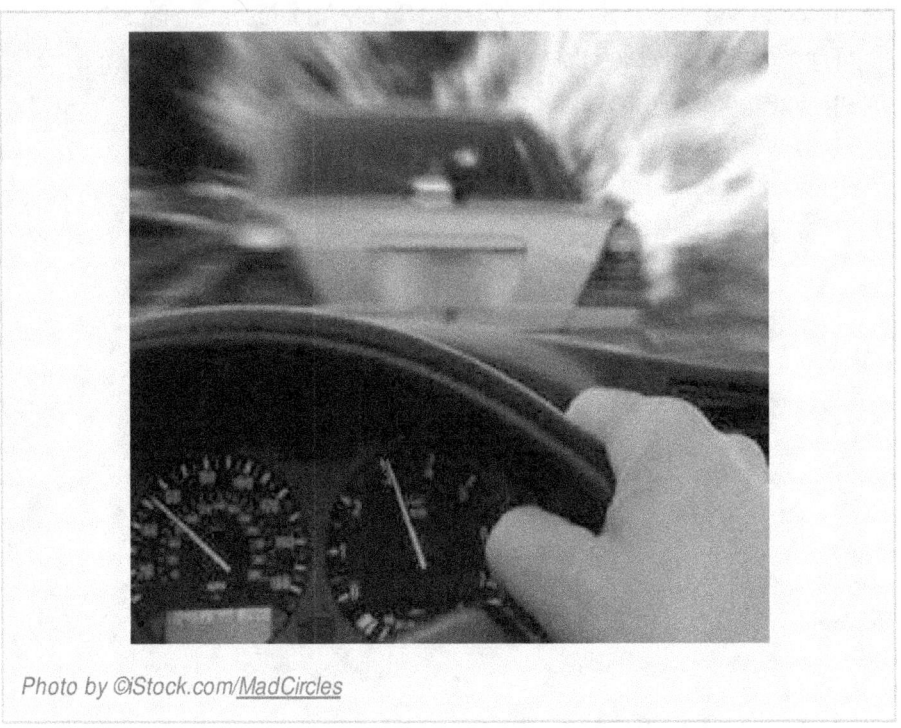

Photo by ©iStock.com/MadCircles

Marijuana significantly impairs judgment, motor coordination, and reaction time, and studies have found a direct relationship between blood THC concentration and impaired driving ability.[7–9]

Marijuana is the illicit drug most frequently found in the blood of drivers who have been involved in vehicle crashes, including fatal ones.[10] Two large European studies found that drivers with THC in their blood were roughly twice as likely to be culpable for a fatal crash than drivers who had not used drugs or alcohol.[11,12] However, the role played by marijuana in crashes is often unclear because it can be detected in body fluids for days or even weeks after intoxication and because people frequently combine it with alcohol. Those involved in vehicle crashes with THC in their blood, particularly higher levels, are three to seven times more likely to be responsible for the incident than drivers who had not used drugs or alcohol. The risk associated with marijuana in combination with alcohol appears to be greater than that for either drug by itself.[8]

Several meta-analyses of multiple studies found that the risk of being involved in a crash significantly increased after marijuana use[13]—in a few cases, the risk doubled or more than doubled.[14–16] However, a large case-control study conducted by the National Highway Traffic Safety Administration found no significant increased crash risk attributable to cannabis after controlling for drivers' age, gender, race, and presence of alcohol.[17]

Is marijuana addictive?

Marijuana use can lead to the development of problem use, known as a marijuana use disorder, which takes the form of addiction in severe cases. Recent data suggest that 30 percent of those who use marijuana may have some degree of marijuana use disorder.[18] People who begin using marijuana before the age of 18 are four to seven times more likely to develop a marijuana use disorder than adults.[19]

Marijuana use disorders are often associated with *dependence*—in which a person feels withdrawal symptoms when not taking the drug. People who use marijuana frequently often report irritability, mood and sleep difficulties, decreased appetite, cravings, restlessness, and/or various forms of physical discomfort that peak within the first week after quitting and last up to 2 weeks.[20,21] Marijuana dependence occurs when the brain adapts to large amounts of the drug by reducing production of and sensitivity to its own endocannabinoid neurotransmitters.[22,23]

Marijuana use disorder becomes addiction when the person cannot stop using the drug even though it interferes with many aspects of his or her life. Estimates of the number of people addicted to marijuana are controversial, in part because epidemiological studies of substance use often use dependence as a proxy for addiction even though it is possible to be dependent without being addicted. Those studies suggest that 9 percent of people who use marijuana will become dependent on it,[24,25] rising to about 17 percent in those who start using in their teens.[26,27]

In 2015, about 4.0 million people in the United States met the diagnostic criteria for a marijuana use disorder;[3] 138,000 voluntarily sought treatment for their marijuana use.[28]

Rising Potency

Marijuana potency, as detected in confiscated samples, has steadily increased over the past few decades.[2] In the early 1990s, the average THC content in confiscated marijuana samples was roughly 3.8 percent. In 2014, it was 12.2 percent. The average marijuana extract contains more than 50 percent THC, with some samples exceeding 80 percent. These trends raise concerns that the consequences of marijuana use could be worse than in the past, particularly among those who are new to marijuana use or in young people, whose brains are still developing (see "What are marijuana's long-term effects on the brain?").

Researchers do not yet know the full extent of the consequences when the body and brain (especially the developing brain) are exposed to high concentrations of THC or whether the recent increases in emergency department visits by people testing positive for marijuana are related to rising potency. The extent to which people adjust for increased potency by using less or by smoking it differently is also unknown. Recent studies suggest that experienced people may adjust the amount they smoke and how much they inhale based on the believed strength of the marijuana they are using, but they are not able to fully compensate for variations in potency.[30,31]

What are marijuana's long-term effects on the brain?

Substantial evidence from animal research and a growing number of studies in humans indicate that marijuana exposure during development can cause long-term or possibly permanent adverse changes in the brain. Rats exposed to THC before birth, soon after birth, or during adolescence show notable problems with specific learning and memory tasks later in life.[32-34] Cognitive impairments in adult rats exposed to THC during adolescence are associated with structural and functional changes in the hippocampus.[35-37] Studies in rats also show that adolescent exposure to THC is associated with an altered reward system, increasing the likelihood that an animal will self-administer other drugs (e.g., heroin) when given an opportunity (see "Is marijuana a gateway drug?").

Imaging studies of marijuana's impact on brain structure in humans have shown conflicting results. Some studies suggest regular marijuana use in adolescence is associated with altered connectivity and reduced volume of specific brain regions involved in a broad range of executive functions such as memory, learning, and impulse control compared to people who do not use.[38,39] Other studies have not found significant structural differences between the brains of people who do and do not use the drug.[40]

Several studies, including two large longitudinal studies, suggest that marijuana use can cause functional impairment in cognitive abilities but that the degree and/or duration of the impairment depends on the age when a person began using and how much and how long he or she used.[41]

Among nearly 4,000 young adults in the Coronary Artery Risk Development in Young Adults study tracked over a 25-year period until mid-adulthood, cumulative lifetime exposure to marijuana was associated with lower scores on a test of verbal memory but did not affect other cognitive abilities such as processing speed or executive function. The effect was sizeable and significant even after eliminating those involved with current use and after adjusting for confounding factors such as demographic factors, other drug and alcohol use, and other psychiatric conditions such as depression.[42]

A large longitudinal study in New Zealand found that persistent marijuana use disorder with frequent use starting in adolescence was associated with a loss of an average of 6 or up to 8 IQ points measured in mid-adulthood.[43] Significantly, in that study, those who used marijuana heavily as teenagers and quit using as adults did not recover the lost IQ points. People who only began using marijuana heavily in adulthood did not lose IQ points. These results suggest that marijuana has its strongest long-term impact on young people whose brains are still busy building new connections and maturing in other ways. The endocannabinoid system is known to play an important role in the proper formation of synapses (the connections between neurons) during early brain development, and a similar role has been proposed for the refinement of neural connections during adolescence. If the long-term effects of marijuana use on cognitive functioning or IQ are upheld by future research, this may be one avenue by which marijuana use during adolescence produces its long-term effects.[44]

However, recent results from two prospective longitudinal twin studies did not support a causal relationship between marijuana use and IQ loss. Those who used marijuana did show a significant decline in verbal ability (equivalent to 4 IQ points) and in general knowledge between the preteen years (ages 9 to 12, before use) and late adolescence/early adulthood (ages 17 to 20). However, at the start of the study, those who would use in the future already had lower scores on these measures than those who would not use in the future, and no predictable difference was found between twins when one used marijuana and one did not. This suggests that observed IQ declines, at least across adolescence, may be caused by shared familial factors (e.g., genetics, family environment), not by marijuana use itself.[45] It should be noted, though, that these studies were shorter in duration than the New Zealand study and did not explore the impact of the dose of marijuana (i.e., heavy use) or the development of a cannabis use disorder; this may have masked a dose- or diagnosis-dependent effect.

The ability to draw definitive conclusions about marijuana's long-term impact on the human brain from past studies is often limited by the fact that study participants use multiple substances, and there is often limited data about the participants' health or mental functioning prior to the study. Over the next decade, the National Institutes of Health is funding the Adolescent Brain

Cognitive Development (ABCD) study—a major longitudinal study that will track a large sample of young Americans from late childhood (before first use of drugs) to early adulthood. The study will use neuroimaging and other advanced tools to clarify precisely how and to what extent marijuana and other substances, alone and in combination, affect adolescent brain development.

Marijuana, Memory, and the Hippocampus

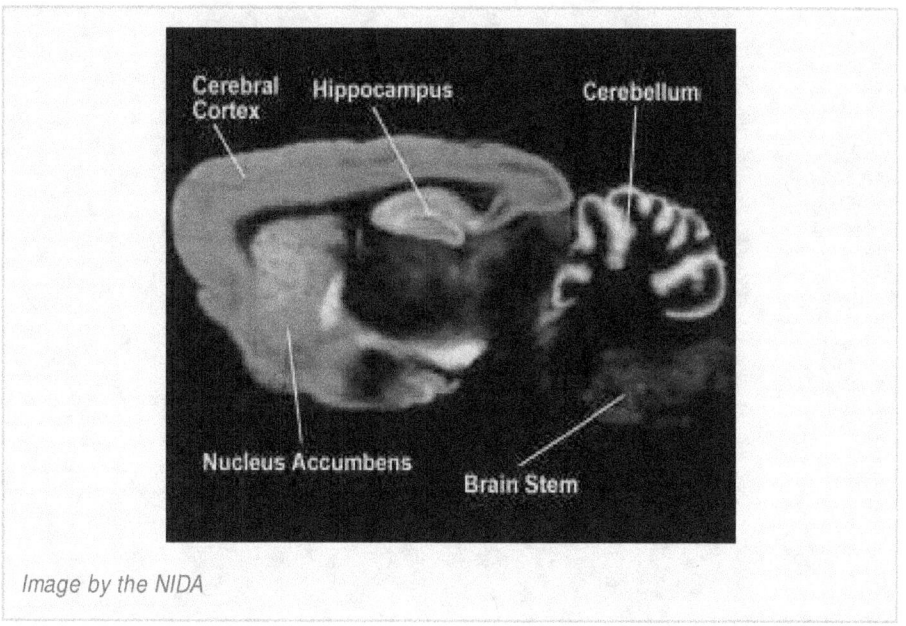

Image by the NIDA

Distribution of cannabinoid receptors in the rat brain. Brain image reveals high levels (shown in orange and yellow) of cannabinoid receptors in many areas, including the cortex, hippocampus, cerebellum, and nucleus accumbens (ventral striatum).

Memory impairment from marijuana use occurs because THC alters how the hippocampus, a brain area responsible for memory formation, processes information. Most of the evidence supporting this assertion comes from animal studies. For example, rats exposed to THC *in utero*, soon after birth, or during adolescence, show notable problems with specific learning/memory tasks later in life. Moreover, cognitive impairment in adult rats is associated with structural and functional changes in the hippocampus from THC exposure during adolescence.

As people age, they lose neurons in the hippocampus, which decreases their ability to learn new information. Chronic THC exposure may hasten age-related loss of hippocampal neurons. In one study, rats exposed to THC every day for 8 months (approximately 30 percent of their lifespan) showed a level of nerve cell loss at 11 to 12 months of age that equaled that of unexposed animals twice their age.

Is marijuana a gateway drug?

Some research suggests that marijuana use is likely to precede use of other licit and illicit substances[46] and the development of addiction to other substances. For instance, a study using longitudinal data from the National Epidemiological Study of Alcohol Use and Related Disorders found that adults who reported marijuana use during the first wave of the survey were more likely than adults who did not use marijuana to develop an alcohol use disorder within 3 years; people who used marijuana and already had an alcohol use disorder at the outset were at greater risk of their alcohol use disorder worsening.[47] Marijuana use is also linked to other substance use disorders including nicotine addiction.

Early exposure to cannabinoids in adolescent rodents decreases the reactivity of brain dopamine reward centers later in adulthood.[48] To the extent that these findings generalize to humans, this could help explain the increased vulnerability for addiction to other substances of misuse later in life that most epidemiological studies have reported for people who begin marijuana use early in life.[49] It is also consistent with animal experiments showing THC's ability to "prime" the brain for enhanced responses to other drugs.[50] For example, rats previously administered THC show heightened behavioral response not only when further exposed to THC but also when exposed to other drugs such as morphine—a phenomenon called *cross-sensitization*.[51]

These findings are consistent with the idea of marijuana as a "gateway drug." However, the majority of people who use marijuana do not go on to use other, "harder" substances. Also, cross-sensitization is not unique to marijuana. Alcohol and nicotine also prime the brain for a heightened response to other drugs[52] and are, like marijuana, also typically used before a person progresses to other, more harmful substances.

It is important to note that other factors besides biological mechanisms, such as a person's social environment, are also critical in a person's risk for drug use. An alternative to the gateway-drug hypothesis is that people who are more vulnerable to drug-taking are simply more likely to start with readily available substances such as marijuana, tobacco, or alcohol, and their subsequent social interactions with others who use drugs increases their chances of trying other drugs. Further research is needed to explore this question.

How does marijuana use affect school, work, and social life?

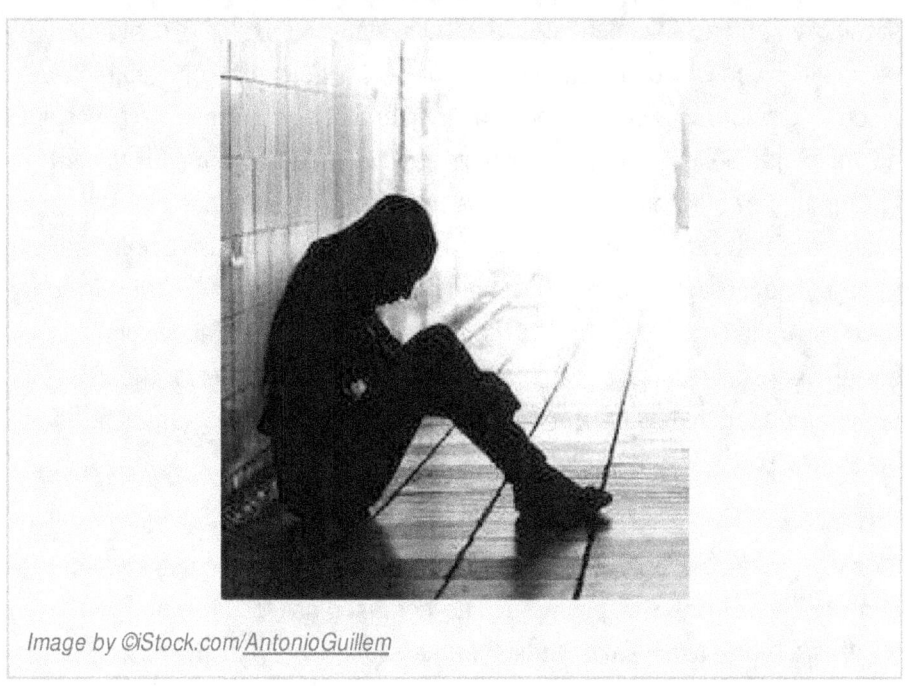

Image by ©iStock.com/AntonioGuillem

Research has shown that marijuana's negative effects on attention, memory, and learning can last for days or weeks after the acute effects of the drug wear off, depending on the person's history with the drug.[53] Consequently, someone who smokes marijuana daily may be functioning at a reduced intellectual level most or all of the time. Considerable evidence suggests that students who smoke marijuana have poorer educational outcomes than their nonsmoking peers. For example, a review of 48 relevant studies found marijuana use to be associated with reduced educational attainment (i.e., reduced chances of graduating).[54] A recent analysis using data from three large studies in Australia and New Zealand found that adolescents who used marijuana regularly were significantly less likely than their non-using peers to finish high school or obtain a degree. They also had a much higher chance of developing dependence, using other drugs, and attempting suicide.[55] Several studies have also linked heavy marijuana use to lower income, greater welfare dependence, unemployment, criminal behavior, and lower life satisfaction.[56,57]

To what degree marijuana use is directly causal in these associations remains an open question requiring further research. It is possible that other factors independently predispose people to both marijuana use and various negative life outcomes such as school dropout.[58] That said, people report a perceived influence of their marijuana use on poor outcomes on a variety of life satisfaction and achievement measures. One study, for example, compared people involved with current and former long-term, heavy use of marijuana with a control group who reported smoking marijuana at least once in their lives but not more than 50 times.[59] All participants had similar education and income backgrounds, but significant differences were found in their educational attainment: Fewer of those who engaged in heavy cannabis use completed college, and more had yearly household incomes of less than $30,000. When asked how marijuana affected their cognitive abilities, career achievements, social lives, and physical and mental health, the majority of those who used heavily reported that marijuana had negative effects in all these areas of their lives.

Studies have also suggested specific links between marijuana use and adverse consequences in the workplace, such as increased risk for injury or accidents.[60] One study among postal workers found that employees who tested positive for marijuana on a pre-employment urine drug test had 55 percent more industrial accidents, 85 percent more injuries, and 75 percent greater absenteeism compared with those who tested negative for marijuana use.[61]

Is there a link between marijuana use and psychiatric disorders?

Several studies have linked marijuana use to increased risk for psychiatric disorders, including psychosis (schizophrenia), depression, anxiety, and substance use disorders, but whether and to what extent it actually causes these conditions is not always easy to determine.[32] The amount of drug used, the age at first use, and genetic vulnerability have all been shown to influence this relationship. The strongest evidence to date concerns links between marijuana use and substance use disorders and between marijuana use and psychiatric disorders in those with a preexisting genetic or other vulnerability.[62]

Research using longitudinal data from the National Epidemiological Survey on Alcohol and Related Conditions examined associations between marijuana use, mood and anxiety disorders, and substance use disorders. After adjusting for various confounding factors, no association between marijuana use and mood and anxiety disorders was found. The only significant associations were increased risk of alcohol use disorders, nicotine dependence, marijuana use disorder, and other drug use disorders.[63]

Recent research (see "AKT1 Gene Variations and Psychosis") has found that people who use marijuana and carry a specific variant of the *AKT1* gene, which codes for an enzyme that affects dopamine signaling in the *striatum*, are at increased risk of developing psychosis. The striatum is an area of the brain that becomes activated and flooded with dopamine when certain stimuli are present. One study found that the risk of psychosis among those with this variant was seven times higher for those who used marijuana daily compared with those who used it infrequently or used none at all.[64]

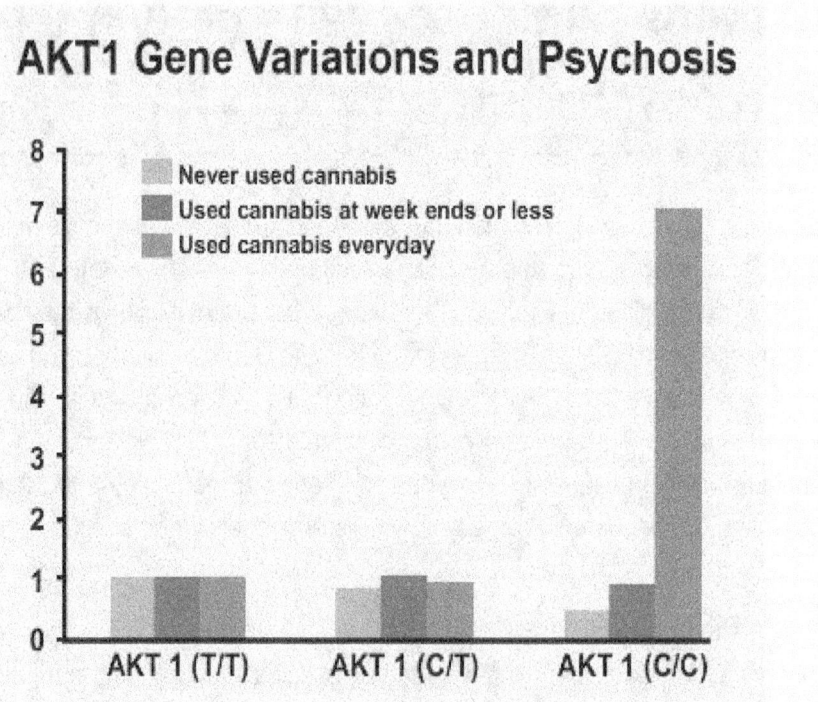

Whether adolescent marijuana use can contribute to developing psychosis later in adulthood appears to depend on whether a person already has a genetically based vulnerability to the disorder. The AKT1 gene governs an enzyme that affects brain signaling involving the neurotransmitter dopamine. Altered dopamine signaling is known to be involved in schizophrenia. AKT1 can take one of three forms in a specific region of the gene implicated in susceptibility to schizophrenia: T/T, C/T, and C/C. Those who use marijuana daily (green bars) with the C/C variant have a seven times higher risk of developing psychosis than those who use it infrequently or use none at all. The risk for psychosis among those with the T/T variant was unaffected by whether they used marijuana.

Source: Di Forti et al. *Biol Psychiatry*. 2012.

Another study found an increased risk of psychosis among adults who had used marijuana in adolescence and also carried a specific variant of the gene for *catechol-O-methyltransferase* (COMT), an enzyme that degrades neurotransmitters such as dopamine and norepinephrine[65] (see "Genetic Variations in COMT Influences the Harmful Effects of Abused Drugs"). Marijuana use has also been shown to worsen the course of illness in patients who already have schizophrenia. As mentioned previously, marijuana can produce an acute psychotic reaction in non-schizophrenic people who use marijuana, especially at high doses, although this fades as the drug wears off.

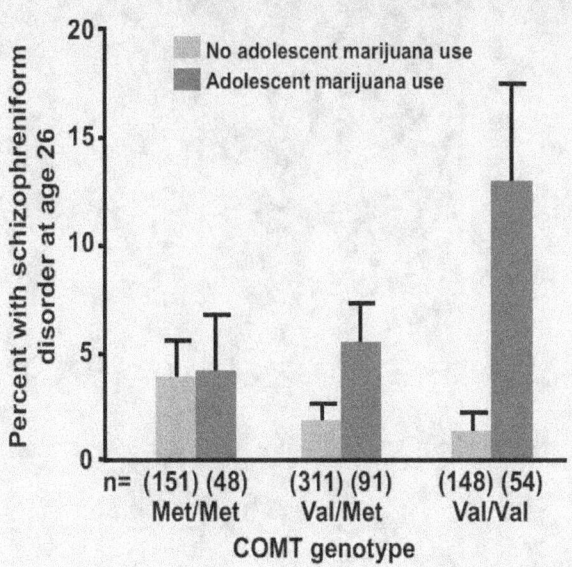

Genetic Variations in COMT Influences the Harmful Effects of Abused Drugs

The influence of adolescent marijuana use on adult psychosis is affected by genetic variables. This figure shows that variations in a gene can affect the likelihood of developing psychosis in adulthood following exposure to cannabis in adolescence. The COMT gene governs an enzyme that breaks down dopamine, a brain chemical involved in schizophrenia. It comes in two forms: "Met" and "Val." Individuals with one or two copies of the Val variant have a higher risk of developing schizophrenic-type disorders if they used cannabis during adolescence (dark bars). Those with only the Met variant were unaffected by cannabis use.

Source: Caspi et al. *Biol Psychiatry*. 2005.

Inconsistent and modest associations have been reported between marijuana use and suicidal thoughts and attempted suicide among teens.[66,67] Marijuana has also been associated with an *amotivational syndrome*, defined as a diminished or absent drive to engage in typically rewarding activities. Because of the role of the endocannabinoid system in regulating mood and reward, it has been hypothesized that brain changes resulting from early use of marijuana may underlie these associations, but more research is needed to verify that such links exist and better understand them.

Adverse Consequences of Marijuana Use

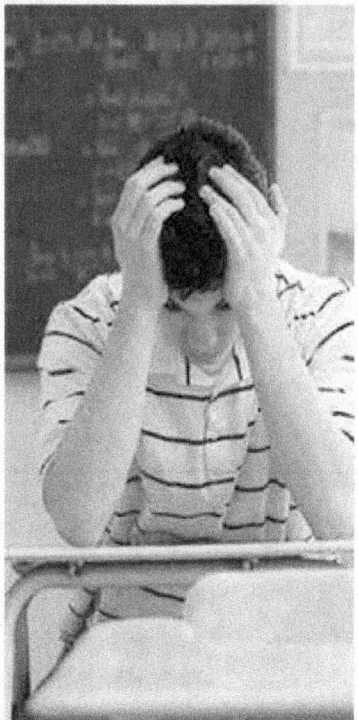

Photo by ©getttyimages.com/Fuse

Acute (present during intoxication)

- Impaired short-term memory
- Impaired attention, judgment, and other cognitive functions
- Impaired coordination and balance
- Increased heart rate
- Anxiety, paranoia
- Psychosis (uncommon)

Persistent (lasting longer than intoxication, but may not be permanent)

- Impaired learning and coordination

- Sleep problems

Long-term (cumulative effects of repeated use)

- Potential for marijuana addiction
- Impairments in learning and memory with potential loss of IQ*
- Increased risk of chronic cough, bronchitis
- Increased risk of other drug and alcohol use disorders
- Increased risk of schizophrenia in people with genetic vulnerability**

Loss of IQ among individuals with persistent marijuana use disorder who began using heavily during adolescence

**These are often reported co-occurring symptoms/disorders with chronic marijuana use. However, research has not yet determined whether marijuana is causal or just associated with these mental problems.*

What are marijuana's effects on lung health?

Like tobacco smoke, marijuana smoke is an irritant to the throat and lungs and can cause a heavy cough during use. It also contains levels of volatile chemicals and tar that are similar to tobacco smoke, raising concerns about risk for cancer and lung disease.[68]

Marijuana smoking is associated with large airway inflammation, increased airway resistance, and lung hyperinflation, and those who smoke marijuana regularly report more symptoms of chronic bronchitis than those who do not smoke.[68,69] One study found that people who frequently smoke marijuana had more outpatient medical visits for respiratory problems than those who do not smoke.[70] Some case studies have suggested that, because of THC's immune-suppressing effects, smoking marijuana might increase susceptibility to lung infections, such as pneumonia, in people with immune deficiencies; however, a large AIDS cohort study did not confirm such an association.[68] Smoking marijuana may also reduce the respiratory system's immune response, increasing the likelihood of the person acquiring respiratory infections, including pneumonia.[69] Animal and human studies have not found that marijuana increases risk for emphysema.[68]

Whether smoking marijuana causes lung cancer, as cigarette smoking does, remains an open question.[68,71] Marijuana smoke contains carcinogenic combustion products, including about 50 percent more benzoprene and 75 percent more benzanthracene (and more phenols, vinyl chlorides, nitrosamines, reactive oxygen species) than cigarette smoke.[68] Because of how it is typically smoked (deeper inhale, held for longer), marijuana smoking leads to four times the deposition of tar compared to cigarette smoking.[72] However, while a few small, uncontrolled studies have suggested that heavy, regular marijuana smoking could increase risk for respiratory cancers, well-designed population studies have failed to find an increased risk of lung cancer associated with marijuana use.[68]

One complexity in comparing the lung-health risks of marijuana and tobacco concerns the very different ways the two substances are used. While people who smoke marijuana often inhale more deeply and hold the smoke in their lungs for a longer duration than is typical with cigarettes, marijuana's effects last longer, so people who use marijuana may smoke less frequently than those who smoke cigarettes.

Additionally, the fact that many people use both marijuana and tobacco makes determining marijuana's precise contribution to lung cancer risk, if any, difficult to establish. Cell culture and animal studies have also suggested THC and CBD may have antitumor effects, and this has been proposed as one reason why stronger expected associations are not seen between marijuana use and lung cancer, but more research is needed on this question.[68]

What are marijuana's effects on other aspects of physical health?

Within a few minutes after inhaling marijuana smoke, a person's heart rate speeds up, the breathing passages relax and become enlarged, and blood vessels in the eyes expand, making the eyes look bloodshot. The heart rate—normally 70 to 80 beats per minute—may increase by 20 to 50 beats per minute or may even double in some cases. Taking other drugs with marijuana can amplify this effect.

Limited evidence suggests that a person's risk of heart attack during the first hour after smoking marijuana is nearly five times his or her usual risk.[73] This observation could be partly explained by marijuana raising blood pressure (in some cases) and heart rate and reducing the blood's capacity to carry oxygen.[74] Marijuana may also cause *orthostatic hypotension* (head rush or dizziness on standing up), possibly raising danger from fainting and falls. Tolerance to some cardiovascular effects often develops with repeated exposure.[75] These health effects need to be examined more closely, particularly given the increasing use of "medical marijuana" by people with health issues and older adults who may have increased baseline vulnerability due to age-related cardiovascular risk factors (see "Is marijuana safe and effective as medicine?").

A few studies have shown a clear link between marijuana use in adolescence and increased risk for an aggressive form of testicular cancer (nonseminomatous testicular germ cell tumor) that predominantly strikes young adult males.[76,77] The early onset of testicular cancers compared to lung and most other cancers indicates that, whatever the nature of marijuana's contribution, it may accumulate over just a few years of use.

Studies have shown that in rare cases, chronic use of marijuana can lead to Cannabinoid Hyperemesis Syndrome—a condition marked by recurrent bouts of severe nausea, vomiting, and dehydration. This syndrome has been found to occur in persons under 50 years of age and with a long history of marijuana use. Cannabinoid Hyperemesis Syndrome can lead sufferers to make frequent trips to the emergency room, but may be resolved when a person stops using marijuana.[78]

Is marijuana safe and effective as medicine?

The potential medicinal properties of marijuana and its components have been the subject of research and heated debate for decades. THC itself has proven medical benefits in particular formulations. The U.S. Food and Drug Administration has approved THC-based medications, dronabinol (Marinol®) and nabilone (Cesamet®), prescribed in pill form for the treatment of nausea in patients undergoing cancer chemotherapy and to stimulate appetite in patients with wasting syndrome due to AIDS.

In addition, several other marijuana-based medications have been approved or are undergoing clinical trials. Nabiximols (Sativex®), a mouth spray that is currently available in the United Kingdom, Canada, and several European countries for treating the spasticity and neuropathic pain that may accompany multiple sclerosis, combines THC with another chemical found in marijuana called cannabidiol (CBD). CBD does not have the rewarding properties of THC, and anecdotal reports indicate it may have promise for the treatment of seizure disorders, among other conditions. A CBD-based liquid medication called Epidiolex is currently being tested in the United States for the treatment of two forms of severe childhood epilepsy, Dravet syndrome and Lennox-Gastaut syndrome.

Researchers generally consider medications like these, which use purified chemicals derived from or based on those in the marijuana plant, to be more promising therapeutically than use of the whole marijuana plant or its crude extracts. Development of drugs from botanicals such as the marijuana plant poses numerous challenges. Botanicals may contain hundreds of unknown, active chemicals, and it can be difficult to develop a product with accurate and consistent doses of these chemicals. Use of marijuana as medicine also poses other problems such as the adverse health effects of smoking and THC-induced cognitive impairment. Nevertheless, a growing number of states have legalized dispensing of marijuana or its extracts to people with a range of medical conditions.

An additional concern with "medical marijuana" is that little is known about the long-term impact of its use by people with health- and/or age-related vulnerabilities—such as older adults or people with cancer, AIDS, cardiovascular disease, multiple sclerosis, or other neurodegenerative diseases. Further research will be needed to determine whether people whose health has been compromised by disease or its treatment (e.g., chemotherapy) are at greater risk for adverse health outcomes from marijuana use.

Medical Marijuana Legalization and Prescription Opioid Use Outcomes

NIDA funded two recent studies that explored the relationship between marijuana legalization and adverse outcomes associated with prescription opioids. The first found an association between medical marijuana legalization and a reduction in overdose deaths from opioid pain relievers, an effect that strengthened in each year following the implementation of legislation.[79] The population-based nature of this study does not establish a causal relationship or give evidence for changes in pain patient behavior.[80,81]

The second NIDA-funded study, a more detailed analysis by the RAND Corporation, showed that legally protected access to medical marijuana dispensaries is associated with lower levels of opioid prescribing, lower self-report of nonmedical prescription opioid use, lower treatment admissions for prescription opioid use disorders, and reduction in prescription opioid overdose deaths.[82] Notably, the reduction in deaths was present only in states with dispensaries (not just medical marijuana laws) and was greater in states with active dispensaries.

Research into the effects of cannabis on opioid use in pain patients is limited, but data suggest that medical cannabis treatment may reduce the dose of opioids required for pain relief.[83,84] In addition to its research portfolio on the roles of the cannabinoid and opioid systems in pain, NIDA is funding additional studies that will provide data relating to medical marijuana and opioids:

- effects of access to medical marijuana on substance use, including nonmedical use of prescription opioids (project numbers DA031816-05, DA039293-01A1, DA037341-02, DA032693-04)

- mental and physical functioning of a cohort of pain patients seeking medical marijuana treatment (DA033397-03)

- the impact of medical marijuana policies on health outcomes (DA034067-03)

Another recent study analyzed Medicare prescription drug coverage data and found that availability of medical marijuana significantly reduced prescribing of medications used for conditions that medical marijuana can treat, including opioids for pain.[85] Overall savings for all prescription drugs were estimated to be $165.2 million in 2013.

Though none of these studies are definitive, they cumulatively suggest that medical marijuana products may have a role in reducing the use of opioids needed to control pain. More research is needed to investigate this possibility.

What are the effects of secondhand exposure to marijuana smoke?

People often ask about the possible psychoactive effect of exposure to secondhand marijuana smoke and whether a person who has inhaled secondhand marijuana smoke could fail a drug test. Researchers measured the amount of THC in the blood of people who do not smoke marijuana and had spent 3 hours in a well-ventilated space with people casually smoking marijuana; THC was present in the blood of the nonsmoking participants, but the amount was well below the level needed to fail a drug test. Another study that varied the levels of ventilation and the potency of the marijuana found that some nonsmoking participants exposed for an hour to high-THC marijuana (11.3 percent THC concentration) in an unventilated room showed positive urine assays in the hours directly following exposure[86]; a follow-up study showed that nonsmoking people in a confined space with people smoking high-THC marijuana reported mild subjective effects of the drug—a "contact high"—and displayed mild impairments on performance in motor tasks.[87]

The known health risks of secondhand exposure to cigarette smoke—to the heart or lungs, for instance—raise questions about whether secondhand exposure to marijuana smoke poses similar health risks. At this point, very little research on this question has been conducted. A 2016 study in rats found that secondhand exposure to marijuana smoke affected a measure of blood vessel function as much as secondhand tobacco smoke, and the effects lasted longer.[88] One minute of exposure to secondhand marijuana smoke impaired flow-mediated dilation (the extent to which arteries enlarge in response to increased blood flow) of the femoral artery that lasted for at least 90 minutes; impairment from 1 minute of secondhand tobacco exposure was recovered within 30 minutes. The effects of marijuana smoke were independent of THC concentration; i.e., when THC was removed, the impairment was still present. This research has not yet been conducted with human subjects, but the toxins and tar levels known to be present in marijuana smoke (see "What are marijuana's effects on lung health?") raise concerns about exposure among vulnerable populations, such as children and people with asthma.

Can marijuana use during and after pregnancy harm the baby?

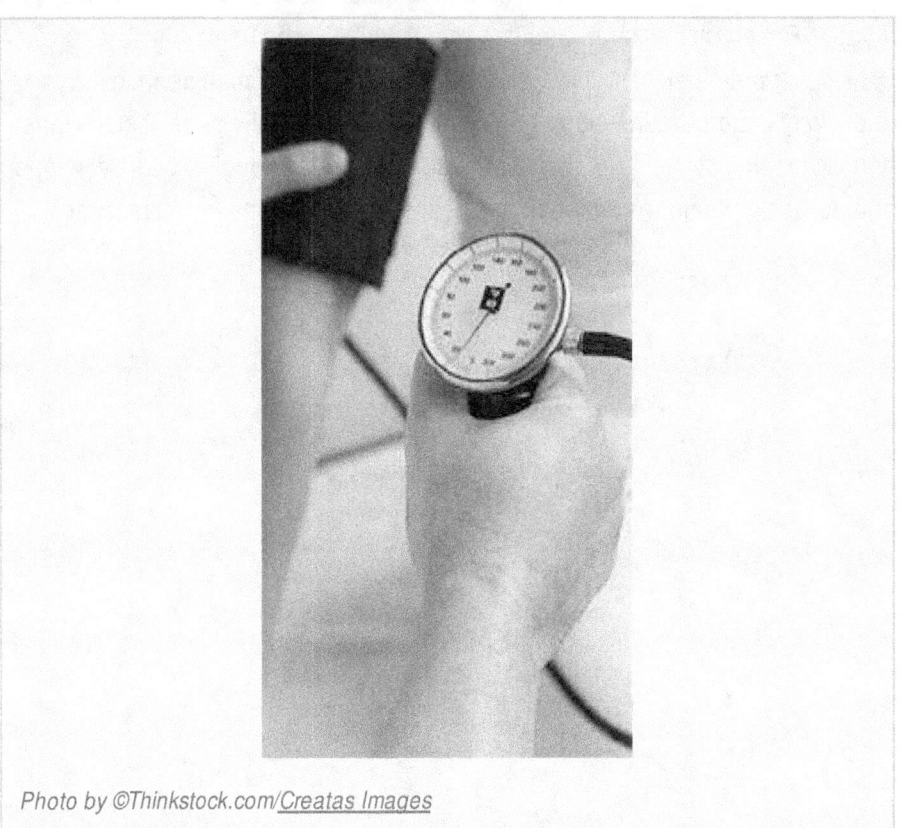

Photo by ©Thinkstock.com/*Creatas Images*

More research is needed on how marijuana use during pregnancy could impact the health and development of infants, given changing policies about access to marijuana, as well as significant increases over the last decade in the number of pregnant women seeking substance use disorder treatment for marijuana use.[89] One study found that about 20% of pregnant women 24-years-old and younger screened positive for marijuana. However, this study also found that women were about twice as likely to screen positive for marijuana use via a drug test than they state in self-reported measures. This suggests that self-reported rates of marijuana use in pregnant females may not be an accurate measure of marijuana use.[90]

There is no human research connecting marijuana use to the chance of miscarriage,[91, 92] although animal studies indicate that the risk for miscarriage increases if marijuana is used early in pregnancy.[93] Some associations have been found between marijuana use during pregnancy and future developmental and hyperactivity disorders in children.[94–97] Evidence is mixed as to whether marijuana use by pregnant women is associated with low birth rate[98–102] or premature birth,[101] although long-term use may elevate these risks.[100] Research has shown that pregnant women who use marijuana have a 2.3 times greater risk of stillbirth.[103] Given the potential of marijuana to negatively impact the developing brain, the American College of Obstetricians and Gynecologists recommends that obstetrician-gynecologists counsel women against using marijuana while trying to get pregnant, during pregnancy, and while they are breastfeeding.[104]

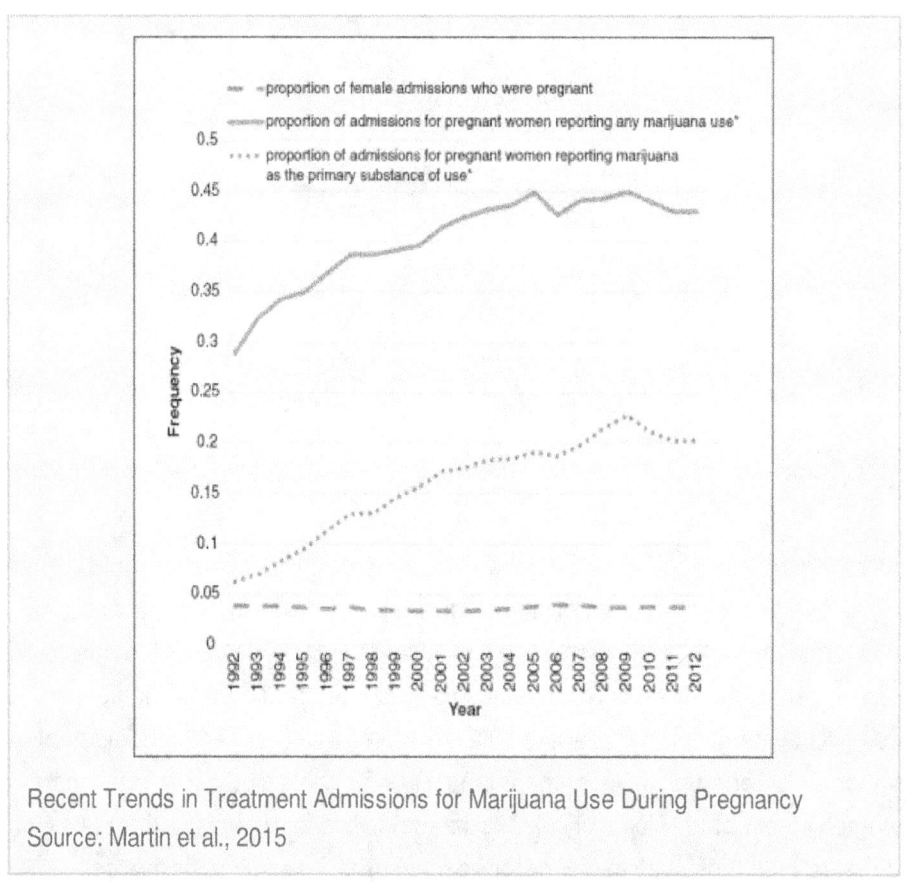

Recent Trends in Treatment Admissions for Marijuana Use During Pregnancy
Source: Martin et al., 2015

Some women report using marijuana to treat severe nausea associated with their pregnancy;[105,106] however, there is no research confirming that this is a safe practice, and it is generally not recommended. Women considering using medical marijuana while pregnant should not do so without checking with their health care providers. Animal studies have shown that moderate concentrations of THC, when administered to mothers while pregnant or nursing, could have long-lasting effects on the child, including increasing stress responsivity and abnormal patterns of social interactions.[107] Animal studies also show learning deficits in prenatally exposed individuals.[33,108]

Human research has shown that some babies born to women who used marijuana during their pregnancies display altered responses to visual stimuli, increased trembling, and a high-pitched cry,[109] which could indicate problems with neurological development.[110] In school, marijuana-exposed children are more likely to show gaps in problem-solving skills, memory,[111] and the ability to remain attentive.[112] More research is needed, however, to disentangle marijuana-specific effects from those of other environmental factors that could be associated with a mother's marijuana use, such as an impoverished home environment or the mother's use of other drugs.[102] Prenatal marijuana exposure is also associated with an increased likelihood of a person using marijuana as a young adult, even when other factors that influence drug use are considered.[113] More information on marijuana use during pregnancy can be found in the NIDA's _Substance Use in Women Research Report_.

Very little is known about marijuana use and breastfeeding. One study suggests that moderate amounts of THC find their way into breast milk when a nursing mother uses marijuana.[114] Some evidence shows that exposure to THC through breast milk in the first month of life could result in decreased motor development at 1 year of age.[115] There have been no studies to determine if exposure to THC during nursing is linked to effects later in the child's life. With regular use, THC can accumulate in human breast milk to high concentrations.[98] Because a baby's brain is still forming, THC consumed in breast milk could affect brain development. Given all these uncertainties, nursing mothers are discouraged from using marijuana.[104,116] New mothers using medical marijuana should be vigilant about coordinating care between the doctor recommending their marijuana use and the pediatrician caring for their baby.

Available Treatments for Marijuana Use Disorders

Marijuana use disorders appear to be very similar to other substance use disorders, although the long-term clinical outcomes may be less severe. On average, adults seeking treatment for marijuana use disorders have used marijuana nearly every day for more than 10 years and have attempted to quit more than six times.[117] People with marijuana use disorders, especially adolescents, often also suffer from other psychiatric disorders (*comorbidity*).[118] They may also use or be addicted to other substances, such as cocaine or alcohol. Available studies indicate that effectively treating the mental health disorder with standard treatments involving medications and behavioral therapies may help reduce marijuana use, particularly among those involved with heavy use and those with more chronic mental disorders. The following behavioral treatments have shown promise:

- **Cognitive-behavioral therapy**: A form of psychotherapy that teaches people strategies to identify and correct problematic behaviors in order to enhance self-control, stop drug use, and address a range of other problems that often co-occur with them.

- **Contingency management**: A therapeutic management approach based on frequent monitoring of the target behavior and the provision (or removal) of tangible, positive rewards when the target behavior occurs (or does not).

- **Motivational enhancement therapy**: A systematic form of intervention designed to produce rapid, internally motivated change; the therapy does not attempt to treat the person, but rather mobilize his or her own internal resources for change and engagement in treatment.

Currently, the FDA has not approved any medications for the treatment of marijuana use disorder, but research is active in this area. Because sleep problems feature prominently in marijuana withdrawal, some studies are examining the effectiveness of medications that aid in sleep. Medications that have shown promise in early studies or small clinical trials include the sleep aid zolpidem (Ambien®), an anti-anxiety/anti-stress medication called buspirone

(BuSpar®), and an anti-epileptic drug called gabapentin (Horizant®, Neurontin®) that may improve sleep and, possibly, executive function. Other agents being studied include the nutritional supplement N-acetylcysteine and chemicals called FAAH inhibitors, which may reduce withdrawal by inhibiting the breakdown of the body's own cannabinoids. Future directions include the study of substances called *allosteric modulators* that interact with cannabinoid receptors to inhibit THC's rewarding effects.

Where can I get further information about marijuana?

To learn more about marijuana and other drugs, visit the NIDA website at **drugabuse.gov** or contact the DrugPubs Research Dissemination Center at 877-NIDA-NIH (877-643-2644; TTY/TDD: 240-645-0228).

The NIDA website includes:

- information about drugs and related health consequences
- NIDA publications, news, and events
- resources for health care professionals
- funding information (including program announcements and deadlines)
- international activities
- links to related websites (access to websites of many other organizations in the field)
- information in Spanish (en español)

NIDA websites and webpages

- drugabuse.gov
- teens.drugabuse.gov
- easyread.drugabuse.gov
- drugabuse.gov/drugs-abuse/marijuana
- drugabuse.gov/related-topics/hivaids
- researchstudies.drugabuse.gov
- irp.drugabuse.gov

For physician information

- NIDAMED: drugabuse.gov/nidamed

Other websites

Information about marijuana is also available through the following websites:

- Substance Abuse and Mental Health Services Administration: samhsa.gov
- Drug Enforcement Administration: dea.gov
- Monitoring the Future: monitoringthefuture.org/
- Partnership for Drug-Free Kids: drugfree.org/drug-guide

This publication is available for your use and may be reproduced **in its entirety** without permission from the NIDA. Citation of the source is appreciated, using the following language: Source: National Institute on Drug Abuse; National Institutes of Health; U.S. Department of Health and Human Services.

References

1. Timberlake DS. A comparison of drug use and dependence between blunt smokers and other cannabis users. *Subst Use Misuse*. 2009;44(3):401-415. doi:10.1080/10826080802347651.

2. Mehmedic Z, Chandra S, Slade D, et al. Potency trends of Δ9-THC and other cannabinoids in confiscated cannabis preparations from 1993 to 2008. *J Forensic Sci*. 2010;55(5):1209-1217. doi:10.1111/j.1556-4029.2010.01441.x.

3. Results from the 2015 National Survey on Drug Use and Health: Detailed Tables, SAMHSA, CBHSQ. http://www.samhsa.gov/data/sites/default/files/NSDUH-DetTabs-2015/NSDUH-DetTabs-2015/NSDUH-DetTabs-2015.htm. Accessed October 11, 2016.

4. Carliner H, Mauro PM, Brown QL, et al. The widening gender gap in marijuana use prevalence in the U.S. during a period of economic change, 2002-2014. *Drug Alcohol Depend*. 2016;170:51-58. doi:10.1016/j.drugalcdep.2016.10.042.

5. Johnston L, O'Malley P, Miech R, Bachman J, Schulenberg J. *Monitoring the Future National Survey Results on Drug Use: 1975-2016: Overview: Key Findings on Adolescent Drug Use.* Ann Arbor, MI: Institute for Social Research, The University of Michigan; 2016.

6. Center for Behavioral Health Statistics and Quality (CBHSQ). *Drug Abuse Warning Network: 2011: Selected Tables of National Estimates of Drug-Related Emergency Department Visits.* Rockville, MD: Substance Abuse and Mental Health Services Administration; 2013.

7. Lenné MG, Dietze PM, Triggs TJ, Walmsley S, Murphy B, Redman JR. The effects of cannabis and alcohol on simulated arterial driving: Influences of driving experience and task demand. *Accid Anal Prev*. 2010;42(3):859-866. doi:10.1016/j.aap.2009.04.021.

8. Hartman RL, Huestis MA. Cannabis effects on driving skills. *Clin Chem*. 2013;59(3):478-492. doi:10.1373/clinchem.2012.194381.

9. Hartman RL, Brown TL, Milavetz G, et al. Cannabis effects on driving lateral control with and without alcohol. *Drug Alcohol Depend*. 2015;154:25-37. doi:10.1016/j.drugalcdep.2015.06.015.

10. Brady JE, Li G. Trends in Alcohol and Other Drugs Detected in Fatally Injured Drivers in the United States, 1999–2010. *Am J Epidemiol*. January 2014:kwt327. doi:10.1093/aje/kwt327.

11. Biecheler M-B, Peytavin J-F, Sam Group, Facy F, Martineau H. SAM survey on "drugs and fatal accidents": search of substances consumed and comparison between drivers involved under the influence of alcohol or cannabis. *Traffic Inj Prev*. 2008;9(1):11-21. doi:10.1080/15389580701737561.

12. *DRUID Final Report: Work Performed, Main Results and Recommendations.* EU DRUID Programme; 2012. http://www.roadsafetyobservatory.com/Evidence/Details/10940.

13. Elvik R. Risk of road accident associated with the use of drugs: a systematic review and meta-analysis of evidence from epidemiological studies. *Accid Anal Prev*. 2013;60:254-267. doi:10.1016/j.aap.2012.06.017.

14. Ramaekers JG, Berghaus G, van Laar M, Drummer OH. Dose related risk of motor vehicle crashes after cannabis use. *Drug Alcohol Depend*. 2004;73(2):109-119.

15. Li M-C, Brady JE, DiMaggio CJ, Lusardi AR, Tzong KY, Li G. Marijuana Use and Motor Vehicle Crashes. *Epidemiol Rev*. 2012;34(1):65-72. doi:10.1093/epirev/mxr017.

16. Asbridge M, Hayden JA, Cartwright JL. Acute cannabis consumption and motor vehicle collision risk: systematic review of observational studies and meta-analysis. *BMJ*. 2012;344:e536. doi:10.1136/bmj.e536.

17. Compton RP, Berning A. *Drug and Alcohol Crash Risk*. Washington, DC: National Highway Traffic Safety Administration; 2015. DOT HA 812 117.

18. Hasin DS, Saha TD, Kerridge BT, et al. Prevalence of Marijuana Use Disorders in the United States Between 2001-2002 and 2012-2013. *JAMA Psychiatry*. 2015;72(12):1235-1242. doi:10.1001/jamapsychiatry.2015.1858.

19. Winters KC, Lee C-YS. Likelihood of developing an alcohol and cannabis use disorder during youth: Association with recent use and age. *Drug Alcohol Depend*. 2008;92(1-3):239-247. doi:10.1016/j.drugalcdep.2007.08.005.

20. Budney AJ, Hughes JR. The cannabis withdrawal syndrome. *Curr Opin Psychiatry*. 2006;19(3):233-238. doi:10.1097/01.yco.0000218592.00689.e5.

21. Gorelick DA, Levin KH, Copersino ML, et al. Diagnostic Criteria for Cannabis Withdrawal Syndrome. *Drug Alcohol Depend*. 2012;123(1-3):141-147. doi:10.1016/j.drugalcdep.2011.11.007.

22. Rotter A, Bayerlein K, Hansbauer M, et al. CB1 and CB2 receptor expression and promoter methylation in patients with cannabis dependence. *Eur Addict Res*. 2013;19(1):13-20. doi:10.1159/000338642.

23. Morgan CJA, Page E, Schaefer C, et al. Cerebrospinal fluid anandamide levels, cannabis use and psychotic-like symptoms. *Br J Psychiatry J Ment Sci*. 2013;202(5):381-382. doi:10.1192/bjp.bp.112.121178.

24. Anthony JC, Warner LA, Kessler RC. Comparative epidemiology of dependence on tobacco, alcohol, controlled substances, and inhalants: Basic findings from the National Comorbidity Survey. *Exp Clin Psychopharmacol*. 1994;2(3):244-268. doi:10.1037/1064-1297.2.3.244.

25. Lopez-Quintero C, Pérez de los Cobos J, Hasin DS, et al. Probability and predictors of transition from first use to dependence on nicotine, alcohol, cannabis, and cocaine: results of the National Epidemiologic Survey on Alcohol and Related Conditions (NESARC). *Drug Alcohol Depend*. 2011;115(1-2):120-130. doi:10.1016/j.drugalcdep.2010.11.004.

26. Anthony JC. The epidemiology of cannabis dependence. In: Roffman RA, Stephens RS, eds. *Cannabis Dependence: Its Nature, Consequences and Treatment*. Cambridge, UK: Cambridge University Press; 2006:58-105.

27. Hall WD, Pacula RL. *Cannabis Use and Dependence: Public Health and Public Policy*. Cambridge, UK: Cambridge University Press; 2003.

28. Center for Behavioral Health Statistics and Quality (CBHSQ). *Treatment Episode Data Set (TEDS): 2003-2013. National Admissions to Substance Abuse Treatment Services*. Rockville, MD: Substance Abuse and Mental Health Services Administration; 2015. BHSIS Series S-75, HHS Publication

No. (SMA) 15-4934.

29. Office of National Drug Control Policy. National Drug Control Strategy: Data Supplement 2015. https://www.whitehouse.gov/sites/default/files/ondcp/policy-and-research/2015_data_supplement_final.pdf. Published 2015. Accessed January 5, 2017.

30. Freeman TP, Morgan CJA, Hindocha C, Schafer G, Das RK, Curran HV. Just say "know": how do cannabinoid concentrations influence users' estimates of cannabis potency and the amount they roll in joints? *Addict Abingdon Engl*. 2014;109(10):1686-1694. doi:10.1111/add.12634.

31. van der Pol P, Liebregts N, Brunt T, et al. Cross-sectional and prospective relation of cannabis potency, dosing and smoking behaviour with cannabis dependence: an ecological study. *Addict Abingdon Engl*. 2014;109(7):1101-1109. doi:10.1111/add.12508.

32. Campolongo P, Trezza V, Cassano T, et al. Perinatal exposure to delta-9-tetrahydrocannabinol causes enduring cognitive deficits associated with alteration of cortical gene expression and neurotransmission in rats. *Addict Biol*. 2007;12(3-4):485-495. doi:10.1111/j.1369-1600.2007.00074.x.

33. Antonelli T, Tomasini MC, Tattoli M, et al. Prenatal exposure to the CB1 receptor agonist WIN 55,212-2 causes learning disruption associated with impaired cortical NMDA receptor function and emotional reactivity changes in rat offspring. *Cereb Cortex N Y N 1991*. 2005;15(12):2013-2020. doi:10.1093/cercor/bhi076.

34. Verrico CD, Gu H, Peterson ML, Sampson AR, Lewis DA. Repeated Δ9-tetrahydrocannabinol exposure in adolescent monkeys: persistent effects selective for spatial working memory. *Am J Psychiatry*. 2014;171(4):416-425. doi:10.1176/appi.ajp.2013.13030335.

35. Rubino T, Realini N, Braida D, et al. Changes in hippocampal morphology and neuroplasticity induced by adolescent THC treatment are associated with cognitive impairment in adulthood. *Hippocampus*. 2009;19(8):763-772. doi:10.1002/hipo.20554.

36. Gleason KA, Birnbaum SG, Shukla A, Ghose S. Susceptibility of the adolescent brain to cannabinoids: long-term hippocampal effects and relevance to schizophrenia. *Transl Psychiatry*. 2012;2:e199.

doi:10.1038/tp.2012.122.

37. Quinn HR, Matsumoto I, Callaghan PD, et al. Adolescent rats find repeated Delta(9)-THC less aversive than adult rats but display greater residual cognitive deficits and changes in hippocampal protein expression following exposure. *Neuropsychopharmacol Off Publ Am Coll Neuropsychopharmacol*. 2008;33(5):1113-1126. doi:10.1038/sj.npp.1301475.

38. Batalla A, Bhattacharyya S, Yücel M, et al. Structural and functional imaging studies in chronic cannabis users: a systematic review of adolescent and adult findings. *PloS One*. 2013;8(2):e55821. doi:10.1371/journal.pone.0055821.

39. Filbey FM, Aslan S, Calhoun VD, et al. Long-term effects of marijuana use on the brain. *Proc Natl Acad Sci U S A*. 2014;111(47):16913-16918. doi:10.1073/pnas.1415297111.

40. Pagliaccio D, Barch DM, Bogdan R, et al. Shared predisposition in the association between cannabis use and subcortical brain structure. *JAMA Psychiatry*. 2015;72(10):994-1001. doi:10.1001/jamapsychiatry.2015.1054.

41. Volkow ND, Swanson JM, Evins AE, et al. Effects of cannabis use on human behavior, including cognition, motivation, and psychosis: a review. *JAMA Psychiatry*. 2016;73(3):292-297. doi:10.1001/jamapsychiatry.2015.3278.

42. Auer R, Vittinghoff E, Yaffe K, et al. Association between lifetime marijuana use and cognitive function in middle age: the Coronary Artery Risk Development in Young Adults (CARDIA) Study. *JAMA Intern Med*. February 2016. doi:10.1001/jamainternmed.2015.7841.

43. Meier MH, Caspi A, Ambler A, et al. Persistent cannabis users show neuropsychological decline from childhood to midlife. *Proc Natl Acad Sci U S A*. 2012;109(40):E2657-E2664. doi:10.1073/pnas.1206820109.

44. Rubino T, Zamberletti E, Parolaro D. Adolescent exposure to cannabis as a risk factor for psychiatric disorders. *J Psychopharmacol Oxf Engl*. 2012;26(1):177-188. doi:10.1177/0269881111405362.

45. Jackson NJ, Isen JD, Khoddam R, et al. Impact of adolescent marijuana use on intelligence: Results from two longitudinal twin studies. *Proc Natl Acad Sci U S A*. 2016;113(5):E500-E508. doi:10.1073/pnas.1516648113.

46. Secades-Villa R, Garcia-Rodríguez O, Jin CJ, Wang S, Blanco C. Probability and predictors of the cannabis gateway effect: a national study. *Int J Drug Policy*. 2015;26(2):135-142. doi:10.1016/j.drugpo.2014.07.011.

47. Weinberger AH, Platt J, Goodwin RD. Is cannabis use associated with an increased risk of onset and persistence of alcohol use disorders? A three-year prospective study among adults in the United States. *Drug Alcohol Depend*. February 2016. doi:10.1016/j.drugalcdep.2016.01.014.

48. Pistis M, Perra S, Pillolla G, Melis M, Muntoni AL, Gessa GL. Adolescent exposure to cannabinoids induces long-lasting changes in the response to drugs of abuse of rat midbrain dopamine neurons. *Biol Psychiatry*. 2004;56(2):86-94. doi:10.1016/j.biopsych.2004.05.006.

49. Agrawal A, Neale MC, Prescott CA, Kendler KS. A twin study of early cannabis use and subsequent use and abuse/dependence of other illicit drugs. *Psychol Med*. 2004;34(7):1227-1237.

50. Panlilio LV, Zanettini C, Barnes C, Solinas M, Goldberg SR. Prior exposure to THC increases the addictive effects of nicotine in rats. *Neuropsychopharmacol Off Publ Am Coll Neuropsychopharmacol*. 2013;38(7):1198-1208. doi:10.1038/npp.2013.16.

51. Cadoni C, Pisanu A, Solinas M, Acquas E, Di Chiara G. Behavioural sensitization after repeated exposure to Delta 9-tetrahydrocannabinol and cross-sensitization with morphine. *Psychopharmacology (Berl)*. 2001;158(3):259-266. doi:10.1007/s002130100875.

52. Levine A, Huang Y, Drisaldi B, et al. Molecular mechanism for a gateway drug: epigenetic changes initiated by nicotine prime gene expression by cocaine. *Sci Transl Med*. 2011;3(107):107ra109. doi:10.1126/scitranslmed.3003062.

53. Schweinsburg AD, Brown SA, Tapert SF. The influence of marijuana use on neurocognitive functioning in adolescents. *Curr Drug Abuse Rev*. 2008;1(1):99-111.

54. Macleod J, Oakes R, Copello A, et al. Psychological and social sequelae of cannabis and other illicit drug use by young people: a systematic review of longitudinal, general population studies. *Lancet Lond Engl*. 2004;363(9421):1579-1588. doi:10.1016/S0140-6736(04)16200-4.

55. Silins E, Horwood LJ, Patton GC, et al. Young adult sequelae of adolescent cannabis use: an integrative analysis. *Lancet Psychiatry*. 2014;1(4):286-293. doi:10.1016/S2215-0366(14)70307-4.

56. Fergusson DM, Boden JM. Cannabis use and later life outcomes. *Addict Abingdon Engl*. 2008;103(6):969-976; discussion 977-978. doi:10.1111/j.1360-0443.2008.02221.x.

57. Brook JS, Lee JY, Finch SJ, Seltzer N, Brook DW. Adult work commitment, financial stability, and social environment as related to trajectories of marijuana use beginning in adolescence. *Subst Abuse*. 2013;34(3):298-305. doi:10.1080/08897077.2013.775092.

58. McCaffrey DF, Pacula RL, Han B, Ellickson P. Marijuana Use and High School Dropout: The Influence of Unobservables. *Health Econ*. 2010;19(11):1281-1299. doi:10.1002/hec.1561.

59. Gruber AJ, Pope HG, Hudson JI, Yurgelun-Todd D. Attributes of long-term heavy cannabis users: a case-control study. *Psychol Med*. 2003;33(8):1415-1422.

60. Macdonald S, Hall W, Roman P, Stockwell T, Coghlan M, Nesvaag S. Testing for cannabis in the work-place: a review of the evidence. *Addict Abingdon Engl*. 2010;105(3):408-416. doi:10.1111/j.1360-0443.2009.02808.x.

61. Zwerling C, Ryan J, Orav EJ. The efficacy of preemployment drug screening for marijuana and cocaine in predicting employment outcome. *JAMA*. 1990;264(20):2639-2643.

62. Radhakrishnan R, Wilkinson ST, D'Souza DC. Gone to Pot - A Review of the Association between Cannabis and Psychosis. *Front Psychiatry*. 2014;5:54. doi:10.3389/fpsyt.2014.00054.

63. Blanco C, Hasin DS, Wall MM, et al. Cannabis Use and Risk of Psychiatric Disorders: Prospective Evidence From a US National Longitudinal Study. *JAMA Psychiatry*. February 2016. doi:10.1001/jamapsychiatry.2015.3229.

64. Di Forti M, Iyegbe C, Sallis H, et al. Confirmation that the AKT1 (rs2494732) genotype influences the risk of psychosis in cannabis users. *Biol Psychiatry*. 2012;72(10):811-816. doi:10.1016/j.biopsych.2012.06.020.

65. Caspi A, Moffitt TE, Cannon M, et al. Moderation of the effect of adolescent-onset cannabis use on adult psychosis by a functional polymorphism in the catechol-O-methyltransferase gene: longitudinal evidence of a gene X environment interaction. *Biol Psychiatry*. 2005;57(10):1117-1127. doi:10.1016/j.biopsych.2005.01.026.

66. Delforterie MJ, Lynskey MT, Huizink AC, et al. The relationship between cannabis involvement and suicidal thoughts and behaviors. *Drug Alcohol Depend*. 2015;150:98-104. doi:10.1016/j.drugalcdep.2015.02.019.

67. Borges G, Bagge CL, Orozco R. A literature review and meta-analyses of cannabis use and suicidality. *J Affect Disord*. 2016;195:63-74. doi:10.1016/j.jad.2016.02.007.

68. Tashkin DP. Effects of marijuana smoking on the lung. *Ann Am Thorac Soc*. 2013;10(3):239-247. doi:10.1513/AnnalsATS.201212-127FR.

69. Owen KP, Sutter ME, Albertson TE. Marijuana: respiratory tract effects. *Clin Rev Allergy Immunol*. 2014;46(1):65-81. doi:10.1007/s12016-013-8374-y.

70. Polen MR, Sidney S, Tekawa IS, Sadler M, Friedman GD. Health care use by frequent marijuana smokers who do not smoke tobacco. *West J Med*. 1993;158(6):596-601.

71. Hashibe M, Morgenstern H, Cui Y, et al. Marijuana use and the risk of lung and upper aerodigestive tract cancers: results of a population-based case-control study. *Cancer Epidemiol Biomark Prev Publ Am Assoc Cancer Res Cosponsored Am Soc Prev Oncol*. 2006;15(10):1829-1834. doi:10.1158/1055-9965.EPI-06-0330.

72. Hancox RJ, Poulton R, Ely M, et al. Effects of cannabis on lung function: a population-based cohort study. *Eur Respir J*. 2010;35(1):42-47. doi:10.1183/09031936.00065009.

73. Mittleman MA, Lewis RA, Maclure M, Sherwood JB, Muller JE. Triggering Myocardial Infarction by Marijuana. *Circulation*. 2001;103(23):2805-2809. doi:10.1161/01.CIR.103.23.2805.

74. Thomas G, Kloner RA, Rezkalla S. Adverse cardiovascular, cerebrovascular, and peripheral vascular effects of marijuana inhalation: what cardiologists need to know. *Am J Cardiol*. 2014;113(1):187-190. doi:10.1016/j.amjcard.2013.09.042.

75. Jones RT. Cardiovascular system effects of marijuana. *J Clin Pharmacol.* 2002;42(11 Suppl):58S - 63S.

76. Lacson JCA, Carroll JD, Tuazon E, Castelao EJ, Bernstein L, Cortessis VK. Population-based case-control study of recreational drug use and testis cancer risk confirms an association between marijuana use and nonseminoma risk. *Cancer.* 2012;118(21):5374-5383. doi:10.1002/cncr.27554.

77. Daling JR, Doody DR, Sun X, et al. Association of marijuana use and the incidence of testicular germ cell tumors. *Cancer.* 2009;115(6):1215-1223. doi:10.1002/cncr.24159.

78. Galli JA, Sawaya RA, Friedenberg FK. Cannabinoid Hyperemesis Syndrome. *Curr Drug Abuse Rev.* 2011;4(4):241-249.

79. Bachhuber MA, Saloner B, Cunningham CO, Barry CL. Medical cannabis laws and opioid analgesic overdose mortality in the United States, 1999-2010. *JAMA Intern Med.* 2014;174(10):1668-1673. doi:10.1001/jamainternmed.2014.4005.

80. Finney JW, Humphreys K, Harris AHS. What ecologic analyses cannot tell us about medical marijuana legalization and opioid pain medication mortality. *JAMA Intern Med.* 2015;175(4):655-656. doi:10.1001/jamainternmed.2014.8006.

81. Bachhuber MA, Saloner B, Barry CL. What ecologic analyses cannot tell us about medical marijuana legalization and opioid pain medication mortality —reply. *JAMA Intern Med.* 2015;175(4):656-657. doi:10.1001/jamainternmed.2014.8027.

82. Powell D, Pacula RL, Jacobson M. *Do Medical Marijuana Laws Reduce Addiction and Deaths Related to Pain Killers?* RAND Corporation; 2015. http://www.rand.org/content/dam/rand/pubs/working_papers/WR1100/WR1130/RAND Accessed April 6, 2017.

83. Abrams DI, Couey P, Shade SB, Kelly ME, Benowitz NL. Cannabinoid-opioid interaction in chronic pain. *Clin Pharmacol Ther.* 2011;90(6):844-851. doi:10.1038/clpt.2011.188.

84. Lynch ME, Clark AJ. Cannabis reduces opioid dose in the treatment of chronic non-cancer pain. *J Pain Symptom Manage.* 2003;25(6):496-498.

85. Bradford AC, Bradford WD. Medical Marijuana Laws Reduce Prescription Medication Use In Medicare Part D. *Health Aff Proj Hope*. 2016;35(7):1230-1236. doi:10.1377/hlthaff.2015.1661.

86. Röhrich J, Schimmel I, Zörntlein S, et al. Concentrations of delta9-tetrahydrocannabinol and 11-nor-9-carboxytetrahydrocannabinol in blood and urine after passive exposure to Cannabis smoke in a coffee shop. *J Anal Toxicol*. 2010;34(4):196-203.

87. Cone EJ, Bigelow GE, Herrmann ES, et al. Non-smoker exposure to secondhand cannabis smoke. I. Urine screening and confirmation results. *J Anal Toxicol*. 2015;39(1):1-12. doi:10.1093/jat/bku116.

88. Wang X, Derakhshandeh R, Liu J, et al. One Minute of Marijuana Secondhand Smoke Exposure Substantially Impairs Vascular Endothelial Function. *J Am Heart Assoc*. 2016;5(8). doi:10.1161/JAHA.116.003858.

89. Martin CE, Longinaker N, Mark K, Chisolm MS, Terplan M. Recent trends in treatment admissions for marijuana use during pregnancy. *J Addict Med*. 2015;9(2):99-104. doi:10.1097/ADM.0000000000000095.

90. Young-Wolff KC, Tucker L-Y, Alexeeff S, et al. Trends in Self-reported and Biochemically Tested Marijuana Use Among Pregnant Females in California From 2009-2016. *JAMA*. 2017;318(24):2490. doi:10.1001/jama.2017.17225

91. Kline J, Hutzler M, Levin B, Stein Z, Susser M, Warburton D. Marijuana and spontaneous abortion of known karyotype. *Paediatr Perinat Epidemiol*. 1991;5(3):320-332.

92. Wilcox AJ, Weinberg CR, Baird DD. Risk factors for early pregnancy loss. *Epidemiol Camb Mass*. 1990;1(5):382-385.

93. Asch RH, Smith CG. Effects of delta 9-THC, the principal psychoactive component of marijuana, during pregnancy in the rhesus monkey. *J Reprod Med*. 1986;31(12):1071-1081.

94. Campolongo P, Trezza V, Ratano P, Palmery M, Cuomo V. Developmental consequences of perinatal cannabis exposure: behavioral and neuroendocrine effects in adult rodents. *Psychopharmacology (Berl)*. 2011;214(1):5-15. doi:10.1007/s00213-010-1892-x.

95. Fried PA, Watkinson B, Gray R. A follow-up study of attentional behavior in 6-year-old children exposed prenatally to marihuana, cigarettes, and alcohol. *Neurotoxicol Teratol*. 1992;14(5):299-311.

96. Goldschmidt L, Day NL, Richardson GA. Effects of prenatal marijuana exposure on child behavior problems at age 10. *Neurotoxicol Teratol*. 2000;22(3):325-336.

97. Fried PA, Smith AM. A literature review of the consequences of prenatal marihuana exposure. An emerging theme of a deficiency in aspects of executive function. *Neurotoxicol Teratol*. 2001;23(1):1-11.

98. Janisse JJ, Bailey BA, Ager J, Sokol RJ. Alcohol, tobacco, cocaine, and marijuana use: relative contributions to preterm delivery and fetal growth restriction. *Subst Abuse*. 2014;35(1):60-67. doi:10.1080/08897077.2013.804483.

99. Hayatbakhsh MR, Flenady VJ, Gibbons KS, et al. Birth outcomes associated with cannabis use before and during pregnancy. *Pediatr Res*. 2012;71(2):215-219. doi:10.1038/pr.2011.25.

100. Shiono PH, Klebanoff MA, Nugent RP, et al. The impact of cocaine and marijuana use on low birth weight and preterm birth: a multicenter study. *Am J Obstet Gynecol*. 1995;172(1 Pt 1):19-27.

101. Mark K, Desai A, Terplan M. Marijuana use and pregnancy: prevalence, associated characteristics, and birth outcomes. *Arch Womens Ment Health*. 2016;19(1):105-111. doi:10.1007/s00737-015-0529-9.

102. Schempf AH, Strobino DM. Illicit Drug Use and Adverse Birth Outcomes: Is It Drugs or Context? *J Urban Health Bull N Y Acad Med*. 2008;85(6):858-873. doi:10.1007/s11524-008-9315-6.

103. Tobacco, drug use in pregnancy can double risk of stillbirth. https://www.nichd.nih.gov/news/releases/Pages/121113-stillbirth-drug-use.aspx. Accessed December 16, 2016.

104. Marijuana Use During Pregnancy and Lactation - ACOG. ACOG. http://www.acog.org/Resources-And-Publications/Committee-Opinions/Committee-on-Obstetric-Practice/Marijuana-Use-During-Pregnancy-and-Lactation. Published July 2015. Accessed October 12, 2016.

105. Roberson EK, Patrick WK, Hurwitz EL. Marijuana use and maternal experiences of severe nausea during pregnancy in Hawai'i. *Hawaii J Med Public Health J Asia Pac Med Public Health*. 2014;73(9):283-287.

106. Westfall RE, Janssen PA, Lucas P, Capler R. Survey of medicinal cannabis use among childbearing women: patterns of its use in pregnancy and retroactive self-assessment of its efficacy against "morning sickness." *Complement Ther Clin Pract*. 2006;12(1):27-33. doi:10.1016/j.ctcp.2005.09.006.

107. Trezza V, Campolongo P, Cassano T, et al. Effects of perinatal exposure to delta-9-tetrahydrocannabinol on the emotional reactivity of the offspring: a longitudinal behavioral study in Wistar rats. *Psychopharmacology (Berl)*. 2008;198(4):529-537. doi:10.1007/s00213-008-1162-3.

108. Mereu G, Fà M, Ferraro L, et al. Prenatal exposure to a cannabinoid agonist produces memory deficits linked to dysfunction in hippocampal long-term potentiation and glutamate release. *Proc Natl Acad Sci U S A*. 2003;100(8):4915-4920. doi:10.1073/pnas.0537849100.

109. Fried PA, Makin JE. Neonatal behavioural correlates of prenatal exposure to marihuana, cigarettes and alcohol in a low risk population. *Neurotoxicol Teratol*. 1987;9(1):1-7.

110. de Moraes Barros MC, Guinsburg R, Mitsuhiro S, Chalem E, Laranjeira RR. Neurobehavioral profile of healthy full-term newborn infants of adolescent mothers. *Early Hum Dev*. 2008;84(5):281-287. doi:10.1016/j.earlhumdev.2007.07.001.

111. Richardson GA, Ryan C, Willford J, Day NL, Goldschmidt L. Prenatal alcohol and marijuana exposure: effects on neuropsychological outcomes at 10 years. *Neurotoxicol Teratol*. 2002;24(3):309-320.

112. Goldschmidt L, Day NL, Richardson GA. Effects of prenatal marijuana exposure on child behavior problems at age 10. *Neurotoxicol Teratol*. 2000;22(3):325-336.

113. Sonon KE, Richardson GA, Cornelius JR, Kim KH, Day NL. Prenatal marijuana exposure predicts marijuana use in young adulthood. *Neurotoxicol Teratol*. 2015;47:10-15. doi:10.1016/j.ntt.2014.11.003.

114. Perez-Reyes M, Wall ME. Presence of delta9-tetrahydrocannabinol in

human milk. *N Engl J Med*. 1982;307(13):819-820. doi:10.1056/NEJM198209233071311.

115. Astley SJ, Little RE. Maternal marijuana use during lactation and infant development at one year. *Neurotoxicol Teratol*. 1990;12(2):161-168.

116. Djulus J, Moretti M, Koren G. Marijuana use and breastfeeding. *Can Fam Physician Médecin Fam Can*. 2005;51:349-350.

117. Budney AJ, Roffman R, Stephens RS, Walker D. Marijuana Dependence and Its Treatment. *Addict Sci Clin Pract*. 2007;4(1):4-16.

118. Diamond G, Panichelli-Mindel SM, Shera D, Dennis M, Tims F, Ungemack J. Psychiatric Syndromes in Adolescents with Marijuana Abuse and Dependency in Outpatient Treatment. *J Child Adolesc Subst Abuse*. 2006;15(4):37-54. doi:10.1300/J029v15n04_02.

www.ingramcontent.com/pod-product-compliance
Lightning Source LLC
Chambersburg PA
CBHW080423240526
45472CB00022B/2234